Dash Diet Cookbook

26 Quick and Easy Recipes

Disclaimer and Terms of Use:

Effort has been made to ensure that the information in this book is accurate and complete, however, the author and the publisher do not warrant the accuracy of the information, text and graphics contained within the book due to the rapidly changing nature of science, research, known and unknown facts and internet. The Author and the publisher do not hold any responsibility for errors, omissions or contrary interpretation of the subject matter herein. This book is presented solely for motivational and informational purposes only.

Table of Contents

Introduction

DASH diet is a well-balanced way of eating different great food choices. The recipes in this guide focus on whole ingredients that are fresh so the transitioning to DASH can be easier. This cookbook would be great for those who are enthusiastic about DASH. These fresh, flavorful recipes are not just for one person who wants to try the DASH way but they are also great for the entire family. Essentially, it is designed for busy individuals but do not want to suffer the consequences of eating high-cholesterol, rich-in-fat foods.

Energize yourself with these recipes that you can follow for quick breakfast, smoothie drink for lunch or healthy dinner. Although these are DASH recipes, they do not mean you have to let go of your favorite foods. If you crave for pasta, then you would be happy to know that we have included quite a few in this list of recipes. Overall, they are DASH-friendly food that can satisfy your cravings.

1. Baked Oatmeal with Blueberries Spice

What You'll Need:

1 whole beaten egg

½ cup of sweetened blueberry sauce

1 ½ cups of non-fat milk

1 tsp vanilla

2 tbsp oil (preferably almond oil)

1 ½ cups of blueberries

2 cups of oats

1 tsp baking powder

¼ tsp salt

1 tsp cinnamon

2 tbsp brown sugar

2 tbsp chopped nuts

How To Prepare:

1. Prepare oven by preheating it to 375ºF (190ºC).

2. Oil the baking pan

3. Mix egg, blueberry sauce, vanilla, oil, milk and blueberries.

4. Get a separate bowl and add in the oats, baking powder, cinnamon and salt.

5. Add it to the liquid ingredients.

6. Mix them well before pouring it into the baking pan.

7. Bake for 25 minutes.

8. Remove it from the oven.

9. Sprinkle the baked oatmeal with brown sugar and nuts.

10. Broil it for 3 to 4 minutes, or until the top is browned. Serve it warm.

Serving Size: 9

2. Frittata

What You'll Need:

6 whole eggs

¼ cup onion (sliced)

1 cup sweet corn (frozen)

1 cup grape-sized tomatoes (cut them in half)

1 cup pepper strips (slice them)

2 tbsp canola oil

1 tsp dry basil

4 oz cheese

How To Prepare:

1. Stir the eggs while you add basil

2. Pour the canola oil into a non-stick pan

3. Heat it before adding the pepper, onion and sweet corn

4. Sauté for 3 minutes

5. Add tomatoes while continue stirring and turning over

6. Cook for 5 minutes or until onions become translucent

7. Add the egg and basil mixture to the pan

8. Allow the egg mixture to fall to the bottom

9. Top it with cheese when the mixture is thickened

10. Use broiler machine to brown the frittata for 3 minutes

Serving Size: 6

3. Blueberry with Greens
What You'll Need:

2 cups mixture of green vegetables (e.g. kale, mustard greens, spinach, collard greens)

4 ice cubes

¼ cup of water

¼ cup of almond milk (unsweetened)

1/3 cup carrot (chopped)

½ cup blueberries (frozen)

½ cup cucumber (chopped but unpeeled)

How To Prepare:

1. Put all the green ingredients in a blender

2. Add water

3. Blend them on low

4. Increase speed to medium when the greens are starting to break down

5. Add the remaining ingredients

6. Blend them all to a high speed for 1 minute or until the desired consistency is achieved.

Serving Size: 2

4. Muffin Sandwich

What You'll Need:

1 ½ tsp scallion (finely chopped, green part only)

1 Swiss cheese (torn to fit into the muffin, reduced fat)

½ English muffin (whole wheat)

½ liquid egg substitute (seasoned)

Olive oil (should be in a pump sprayer)

How To Prepare:

1. Toast the muffin for about a minute or two

2. Turn off the toaster and top the muffin with the cheese

3. Allow it to stand for 30 seconds

4. Transfer to a bowl or a plate

5. Spray a skillet with oil

6. Heat it over medium heat.

7. Add the egg and cook for 15 seconds or until its edges are set

8. Lift its edges to allow the uncooked liquid to flow underneath

9. Continue lifting and cooking its edges every 15 seconds

10. Fold the egg mixture's edges into the center to create a patty-like shape.

11. Transfer it to the muffin

12. Sprinkle with scallion

13. Serve

Serving Size: 1

5. Open-faced Sandwich with Strawberries

What You'll Need:

1 bread (sliced, whole-grain)

2 tbsp cream cheese (fat-free)

2 strawberries (hulled and sliced)

1 tsp honey (optional)

How To Prepare:

1. Toast the bread using a toaster or broiler for one to two minutes.

2. Spread cream cheese

3. Top it with strawberries

4. Drizzle with honey (if you wish)

Serving Size: 1

6. Almond Butter and Banana

What You'll Need:

2 slices of bread (100% whole wheat)

2 tbsp almond butter

1 banana (sliced

1/8 tsp cinnamon (ground)

How To Prepare:

1. Toast the bread

2. Spread each sliced bread with butter

3. Place sliced banana on top

4. Sprinkle it with cinnamon

Serving Size: 1

7. Bowl of Protein

What You'll Need:

1 tbsp almond butter

½ banana (medium-sized, thinly sliced)

¾ cup cottage cheese (low-fat)

¼ cup oats

How To Prepare:

1. Mix all ingredients in a bowl

2. Serve

Serving Size: 1

8. Chicken Breasts with Salad
What You'll Need:

For the salad, prepare the following:

Cracked black pepper

1 cup cherry tomatoes

2 zucchini (small size, thinly sliced, cut into half moons)

4 cups arugula

1 cup mozzarella cheese (fresh, diced)

¼ cup olive oil (extra virgin)

¼ cup vinegar (balsamic)

2 tbsp fresh basil (chopped)

1/8 tsp sea salt

How to Prepare:

1. Combine tomatoes, zucchini, cheese in a bowl

2. Add the oil, salt, pepper and vinegar to taste

3. Mix them well

4. Refrigerate until the chicken is already prepared

For the Chicken

Cracked black pepper

4 chicken breasts (boneless, skinless)

1 tsp dried oregano

½ tsp rosemary (minced, fresh)

½ tsp garlic powder

1/8 tsp sea salt

How To Prepare:

1. Take the fat off the chicken breasts

2. Mix the oregano, rosemary, salt, pepper, and garlic powder to taste

3. Sprinkle the mixture on the sides of the chicken

4. Get a large saucepan and heat over medium heat

5. Coat it with olive oil spray

6. Add the chicken when the oil is hot (two at a time)

7. Cook per side for 4 to 6 minutes

8. Remove the salad from the fridge while waiting for the chicken

9. Add the arugula and basil to the salad

10. Toss well

11. Allow the chicken breasts to rest for 2 minutes, once they are done cooking.

12. Slice the breast diagonally to great strips of chicken

13. Top the salad with sliced chicken

Serving Size: 4

9. Almond-Date Shake

What You'll Need:

4 ice cubes

2 tbsp warm water

2 cups almond milk (vanilla flavor and chilled)

1 banana (ripe and frozen)

1/3 cup pitted dates (chopped)

½ cup vanilla soy (fat-free)

1/8 tsp nutmeg (ground)

How To Prepare:

1. Place the dates in a bowl

2. Sprinkle them with warm water

3. Soak for at least 5 minutes until they are softened

4. Drain the water

5. Add the softened dates, almond milk, banana, yogurt, ice cubes, and nutmeg.

6. Blend until smooth and frothy

7. Transfer smoothie to a tall glass

8. Top it with nutmeg

Serving Size: 1 cup

10. Mexican Chicken Soup

What You'll Need for the Soup:

1 tbsp olive oil

1 ½ pounds chicken thighs (boneless, cut into bite-sized)

1 yellow onion (chopped)

1 red bell pepper (cored and cut)

1 zucchini (large, trimmed and cut into dices)

1 jalapeno (seeded and chopped)

3 cups chicken broth (homemade or low-sodium)

3 cups of water

1 tomato juice (no-salt added, un-drained)

2 tbsp cilantro (fresh, chopped)

Lime wedges

How To Prepare the Soup:

1. Heat oil in a large pot over medium-high heat

2. Cook the chicken in two batches

3. Stir occasionally, until they are browned

4. Add onion, red pepper, garlic, zucchini and jalapeno

5. Cook them all until the onion softens

6. Stir in the broth

7. Add the water and tomatoes with juice

8. Bring the mixture to a boil

9. Simmer them until the chicken turns opaque

10. Stir in corn and cilantro

What You'll Need for the Tortilla Chips:

Olive oil

3 corn tortillas (cut in strips)

How to Prepare:

1. Preheat oven to 400° F (204°C).

2. Spray its baking sheet with oil

3. Spread the tortilla strips on the sheet and spray them with oil

4. Bake until crisp and golden brown

5. Remove from oven.

6. Go back to the soup and transfer it to a bowl.

7. Sprinkle each bowl with 1 tbsp of tortilla chips

8. Add cilantro

9. Squeeze lime wedges into the soup

Serving Size: 1 ¼ cups

11. Ground Sirloin with Chili

What You'll Need:

1 tbsp olive oil

1 yellow onion

1 green bell pepper

2 cloves of garlic

1 ¼ pounds ground sirloin

2 tbsp chili powder

½ tsp chili chipotle

½ Kosher salt

28 ounces low-sodium tomatoes

15 ounces pinto beans

Cheddar cheese

Non-fat sour cream

Fresh cilantro

How To Prepare:

1. Heat 1 tbsp olive oil in a saucepan

2. Add 1 medium-sized, chopped yellow onion and 1 cored, chopped medium-sized green bell pepper to the pan

3. Cook and stir for 3 minutes

4. Add 2 cloves of minced garlic for 1 minute or until fragrant

5. Add 1 ¼ pounds ground sirloin and cook

6. Stir in 2 tbsp chili powder, ½ tsp ground, chili chipotle and ½ tsp kosher salt

7. Cook for 1 minute

8. Add 28 ounces of chopped, low-sodium tomatoes with juice

9. Bring to a boil for 15 minutes or until the juice thickened

10. Add 15 ounces of low-sodium well-rinsed pinto beans without the juice for 5 minutes.

11. Add low-fat, shredded cheddar cheese, non-fat sour cream and chopped fresh cilantro leaves, if desired.

Serving Size: 6

12. Beef and Cracked Wheat Meat Loaf

What You'll Need:

1/2 cup cracked wheat

2 tsp canola oil

2 cloves garlic

1 red bell pepper

2 cloves

1 yellow onion

1 tbsp Worcestershire sauce

1 tsp kosher salt

1/2 tsp ground black pepper

2 large egg whites

1 pound ground sirloin

How To Prepare:

1. Mix 1 cup boiling water and ½ cup cracked wheat in a bowl

2. Let the mixture stand for 20 minutes

3. Preheat oven to 350ºF (176ºC)

4. Place aluminum foil over baking sheet and spray with canola oil

5. Heat 2 tsp canola oil in a skillet

6. Add 2 cloves, minced garlic, 1 medium-sized, cored and diced red bell pepper and 2 cloves and 1 medium-sized, minced yellow onion.

7. Cook and stir for 6 minutes.

8. Transfer the mixture to a bowl and allow to cool down.

9. Drain cracked wheat in a sieve

10. Add it to the bowl with the mixture.

11. Stir in ketchup, 1 tbsp Worcestershire sauce, 1 tsp kosher salt and ½ tsp ground black pepper

12. Add 2 large egg whites and 1 pound ground sirloin

13. Shape into loaf using the foil-lined baking sheet

14. Bake until loaf is golden brown

15. Slice and serve

Serving Size: 8

13. Papaya Goodness

What You'll Need:

1 cup spinach,

1 cup kale

1 green apple

1 papaya

1 tbsp ground flaxseed

How To Prepare:

1. Place 1 cup spinach, 1 cup chopped kale, ¾ cup water in a blender

2. Blend on low

3. Add 1 green, coarsely chopped apple, 1 cup coarsely chopped papaya and 1 tbsp ground flaxseed.

4. Blend for 1 minute

5. Serve

Serving Size: 2

14. Quinoa Salad

What You'll Need:

1/4 cup green onion

1 1/2 fresh mint

1/2 cup carrot

1/2 cup red bell pepper

1/8 tsp pepper flakes

1/2 tsp orange zest

2 tbsp Thai basil

1/2 orange juice

1 tsp sesame seeds

1 tbsp sesame oil

1 tbsp extra virgin olive oil

1/8 tsp black pepper

How To Prepare:

1. Rinse quinoa before adding it to a covered pot along with vegetable broth

2. Bring it to a boil

3. Simmer for 15 minutes

4. Remove from heat

5. Transfer it to a bowl

6. Add 1 cup shelled, ¼ cup chopped green onion, 1 ½ tsp fresh, finely chopped mint, ½ cup chopped carrot, ½ cup chopped red bell pepper, 1/8 tsp pepper flakes, ½ tsp orange zest (grated), 2 tbsp fresh, finely chopped Thai basil, ½ cup orange juice, 1 tsp sesame seeds, 1 tbsp sesame oil, 1 tbsp extra virgin olive oil, and 1/8 tsp black pepper.

7. Mix them well before serving.

Serving Size: 6

15. Italian Pasta Salad

What You'll Need:

4 tbsp virgin coconut oil

4 cups whole-wheat penne pasta

2 cups cherry tomatoes

1 cup mozzarella cheese

1 cup basil

Pinch sea salt

1/8 tsp cracked bell pepper

How To Prepare:

1. Boil one to two liters of water in a pot

2. Add 4 tbsp extra virgin coconut oil

3. Add 4 cups whole-wheat penne pasta

4. Cook for 10 minutes

5. Strain the pasta

6. Prepare large pan and heat it over medium-high heat

7. Toast pine nuts for 2 minutes and stir frequently

8. Remove nuts from the pan

9. Toss cooked pasta in a large bowl and add 2 cups cherry tomatoes, 1 cup, chopped mozzarella cheese, 1 cup fresh, coarsely chopped basil, pinch sea salt and 1/8 tsp cracked black pepper.

Serving Size: 4

16. Baked Sunflower Seed

What You'll Need:

6 ounces turkey breast

1 1/2 cups sunflower seeds

2 tbsp parsley

1/4 tsp paprika

1/4 tsp cayenne pepper

1/4 tsp cumin

3 egg whites

How To Prepare:

1. Preheat oven to 400ºF (204ºC).

2. Cut 6 ounces skinless, boneless turkey breast in half

3. Use food processor to combine 1 ½ cups unsalted sunflower seeds, 2 tbsp chopped, fresh parsley, ¼ tsp paprika, ¼ tsp cayenne pepper and ¼ tsp cumin

4. Pour the mixture onto a plate while spread the flour in a separate plate

5. Whisk 3 egg whites in a shallow bowl

6. Dip each breast in a flour plate, egg bowl and seed mixture and place the chicken breasts in the oven

7. Bake for 10 minutes

8. Serve

Serving Size: 4

17. Orange Chicken with Brown Rice

What You'll Need:

1 tbsp sesame oil

1 tbsp olive oil

1/2 cup mushroom

1 minced clove garlic

1/4 cup white onion

4 ounces chicken breasts

1/4 tsp cracked black pepper

1/4 tsp ground ginger

1/4 tsp lemon zest

1/2 tsp orange zest

1/2 cup orange juice

4 cups spinach

How To Prepare:

1. Heat 1 tbsp sesame oil and 1 tbsp olive oil in a pan over high heat

2. Add ½ cup coarsely chopped mushroom, 1 large minced clove garlic, ¼ cup chopped white onion

3. Cook for 1 minute

4. Add 4 ounces skinless chicken breasts and season with ¼ tsp cracked black pepper, 1/4 tsp ground

ginger, ¼ tsp grated lemon zest, and ½ tsp grated orange zest.

5. Cook for 5 minutes

6. Add ½ cup orange juice

7. Stir and add 4 cups spinach

8. Remove it from the heat

9. Divide cooked brown rice into 2 dishes

11. Top it with orange chicken

Serving Size: 4

18. Roasted Plums

What You'll Need:

6 plums

1 tbsp unsalted butter

1 tbsp unsalted butter

1 tbsp sugar

1/2 cup Greek yogurt

2 tbsp nuts

2 tsp honey

How To Prepare:

1. Heat oven to 375°F (190°C).

2. Place parchment paper over a baking sheet

3. Add 6 pitted plums over sheet

4. Brush with 1 tbsp unsalted butter

5. Sprinkle with 1 tbsp sugar

6. Bake for 15 minutes

7. Divide plums into 4 bowls and top each with ½ cup Greek yogurt

8. Sprinkle with 2 tbsp nuts and add 2 tsp honey

Serving Size: 2

19. Fresh Fruit Platter with Sauce

What You'll Need:

1 large mango

2 tbsp water

2tbsp sugar

1 tbsp maple syrup

2 tsp fresh ginger

1 tsp vanilla extract

Fresh fruits of your liking

How To Prepare:

1. Place 1 quartered, large mango, 2 tbsp water, 2 tbsp sugar, 1 tbsp maple syrup, 2 tsp fresh ginger, and 1 tsp vanilla extract to a food processor

2. Transfer mixture into a bowl

3. Serve it with a platter of fresh fruits, such as oranges, kiwi, strawberries, bananas, and cantaloupe.

Serving Size: 6

20. Tomato, Bell Pepper Soup

What You'll Need:

2 1/2 cups tomato juice

11 ounces tomatoes

1/2 cup red bell pepper

2 tbsp extra virgin olive oil

1 tbsp red wine vinegar

1 tbsp white horseradish

1 garlic clove

Hot pepper sauce

How To Prepare:

1. Combine 2 ½ cups tomato juice, 11 ounces finely chopped tomatoes, ½ cup chopped roasted red bell pepper, 2 tbsp extra virgin olive oil, 1 tbsp red wine vinegar, 1 tbsp white horseradish, 1 pressed garlic clove, and hot pepper sauce in a bowl.

2. Mix them well.

3. Season it with sea salt and ground black pepper.

Serving Size: 6

21. Pork Chops in Sauce

What You'll Need:

4 ounces pork loin chops

Cornstarch

Milk

Musk

How To Prepare:

1. Spray skillet with oil and heat it over medium heat

2. Season 4 ounces pork loin chops with salt and pepper

3. Add the pork to the skillet

4. Cook it for 3 minutes

5. Transfer pork to a plate

6. Place cornstarch to a small bowl and add broth

7. Add milk and musk

8. Whisk

9. Melt butter in skillet and add shallots

10. Cook and stir for 1 minute

11. Pour broth mixture in the skillet and bring to a boil

12. Add the pork to the skillet and cook

13. Transfer it to a platter and pour sauce over the pork chops

Serving Size: 4

22. Baked Cajun Catfish

What You'll Need:

3 pieces potatoes

4 pieces bell pepper

1 celery

1 clove garlic

1 cup tomatoes

1 cup scallions

How To Prepare:

1. Preheat oven to 400ºF (204ºC) and spray baking dish with oil

2. Heat a nonstick skillet and add 1 tbsp oil

3. Add potatoes and cook for 5 minutes

4. Add bell pepper, celery and garlic

5. Sauté until pepper softens

6. Add tomatoes and scallions

7. Sprinkle with salt

8. Spread in the baking dish and bake for 25 minutes

9. Remove from the oven and add catfish on vegetable mixture

10. Sprinkle fish with Cajun seasoning

11. Bake for 10 minutes

12. Serve hot

Serving Size: 4

23. Oatmeal with Apple and Cinnamon

What You'll Need:

1 1/2 cups almond milk

1 cup oats

1 large apple

1/4 tsp ground cinnamon

How To Prepare:

1. Heat 1 ½ cups almond milk (unsweetened) and simmer over medium heat before adding 1 cup oats and 1 large, unpeeled and cubed apple.

2. Stir until most liquid is absorbed

3. Add ¼ tsp ground cinnamon and stir

4. Scoop the mixture into two bowls

5. Top with walnuts

Serving Size: 2

24. Homemade Granola

What You'll Need:

3 cups oats

1/4 cup flaxseeds

1 cup almonds

1/2 tsp cinnamon

1/4 tsp ground ginger

1/4 cup brown sugar

1/4 cup maple syrup

1/2 tsp almond extract

1 cup golden raisins

How To Prepare:

1. Preheat oven to 250ºF (121ºC).

2. Combine 3 cups oats, ¼ cup flaxseeds, 1 cup sliced almonds, ½ tsp ground cinnamon, ¼ tsp ground ginger, and ¼ cup brown sugar in a bowl.

3. Mix ¼ cup maple syrup and ½ tsp almond extract.

4. Pour wet ingredients into the dry ingredients or oat mixture and mix well

5. Transfer mixture to sheet pans and bake for 75 minutes

6. Remove from oven and transfer to a bowl

7. Place 1 cup golden raisins evenly

Serving Size: 12

25. Fruity Yogurt

What You'll Need:

Yogurt

1 cup blueberries

1 cup strawberries

1 cup flaxseed

1 Granola

How To Prepare:

1. Scoop yogurt into a parfait dish

2. Top it with blueberries, strawberries, flaxseed meal and granola

3. Layer remaining yogurt and top it with strawberries, blueberries, kiwifruit, flaxseeds and granola.

Serving Size: 1

26. Vinaigrette

What You'll Need:

1/2 tsp brown mustard

1/2 tsp marmalade

1/4 cup red wine vinegar

1/2 cup virgin olive oil

1/8 tsp sea salt

How To Prepare:

1. Combine and whisk ½ tsp brown mustard, ½ tsp low-sugar marmalade and ¼ cup red wine vinegar

2. Drizzle in ½ cup extra virgin olive oil while continue whisking

3. Add 1/8 tsp sea salt and cracked pepper

4. Store in a container if you will not use it immediately

Serving Size: 6

Conclusion

This type of diet is an effective way to lose weight and follow a healthy lifestyle. Let this report guide you in transitioning from a non-healthy diet to a heart-friendly diet. By following the guidelines in this report, you can surely fight off chronic disease and prevent weight gain or achieve weight loss.

The DASH recipes presented here can be your perfect guide in lowering your cholesterol. They are especially great if you are prone to heart disease. These are 25 recipes that you can cook up for a week or two and practice your skills in making a reduced-sodium meal.